I0404193

The Zika Project

By microbiologist and investigative author

Gwendolyn Olmsted

Amazon.com
Seattle, WA, U.S.A.

First published as
The Zika Project
4 August 2016

1. Microbiology 2. Zika 3. Population Control

The Zika Project
Available in paperback and *Kindle* © e-book formats

ISBN-13: 978-1536876390
ISBN-10: 1536876399

SUMMARY

The Zika virus was first discovered in 1947 throughout Africa and southern Asia, so this is nothing new. Eyebrows were raised however, in 2013 when small outbreaks and individual cases were officially documented in Africa, the western pacific, and the Americas. The media reported that "Brazil is now considered the epicenter of the Zika outbreak, which coincides with at least 4,000 reports of babies born with microcephaly just since October:" Microcephaly is a birth defect associated with a shrunken brain.

The World Health Organization stated the Zika virus could potentially pose a bigger threat to global health. With that, the United States called for a massive research effort to develop a vaccine for solutions and future prevention.

The Zika virus had never been a threat to the global population before, so what really happened between 2010 and 2015? Read as the solution unravels with gaining evidence that points in the direction towards the new world order with a new term the leaders of the free world, both private and public, have coined ... DEPOPULATION.

OTHER BOOKS WRITTEN BY THE SAME AUTHOR

The Evolution of Ebola

Eight Weeks in May

The Pity Date

American Cockthief

The *Sidebar* series

Sex in Florida

American Sociopath

Running on the Luck of my Heart:
The Horace Greasley story

Marilyn Monroe: The Live-In Housekeeper Did It

Available at:

Gwendolyn Olmsted's author page on Amazon.com

CONTENTS

12. About the Author

FORWARD

Armageddon, or not......

A thought on my neuron is impinging,
If it ain't Armageddon, do stop whining,
"A happy heart makes a cheerful face,"
A notion apt for our global race,
Smiles to each one are a grace,
Blessing to all as we set our pace,
Way too much negativity.
Largely a waste of futility,
Instead of daily positivity,
Way too much 'stinking thinking',
If it ain't Armageddon, do stop whining,'
This thought on my neuron is impinging.

~Julie Grenness

CHAPTER ONE:
WHAT IS ZIKA VIRUS?

Zika virus (ZIKV) is a member of the virus family *Flaviviridae* and the genus *Flavivirus.*

It is spread by daytime-active *Aedes* mosquitoes, such as *A. aegypti* and *A. albopictus.* Its name comes from the Zika Forest of Uganda, where the virus was first isolated in 1947. Zika virus is related to the dengue, yellow fever, Japanese encephalitis, and West Nile viruses. Since the 1950s, it has been known to occur within a narrow equatorial belt from Africa to Asia.

From 2007 to 2016, the virus spread eastward, across the Pacific Ocean to the Americas, where the 2015–16 Zika virus epidemic has reached pandemic levels.

The infection, known as Zika fever or Zika virus disease, often causes no or only mild symptoms, similar to a very mild form of dengue fever.

As of 2016, the illness cannot be prevented by medications or vaccines. Zika can also spread from a pregnant woman to her fetus. This can result in microcephaly, severe brain malformations, and other birth defects. Zika infections in adults may result rarely in Guillain–Barré syndrome.

In January 2016, the United States Centers for Disease Control and Prevention issued travel guidance on affected countries, including the use of enhanced precautions, and guidelines for pregnant women including considering postponing travel. Other governments or health agencies also issued similar travel warnings, while Colombia, the Dominican Republic, Ecuador, El Salvador, and Jamaica advised women to postpone getting pregnant until more is known about the disease.

Virology: The Zika virus belongs to the *Flaviviridae* family and the *Flavivirus* genus, and is thus related to the dengue, yellow fever, Japanese encephalitis, and West Nile viruses. Like other flaviviruses, Zika virus is enveloped andicosahedral and has a nonsegmented, single-stranded, 10 kilobase positive-sense RNA genome. It is most closely related to the Spondweni virus and is one of the two viruses in the Spondweni virus clade.

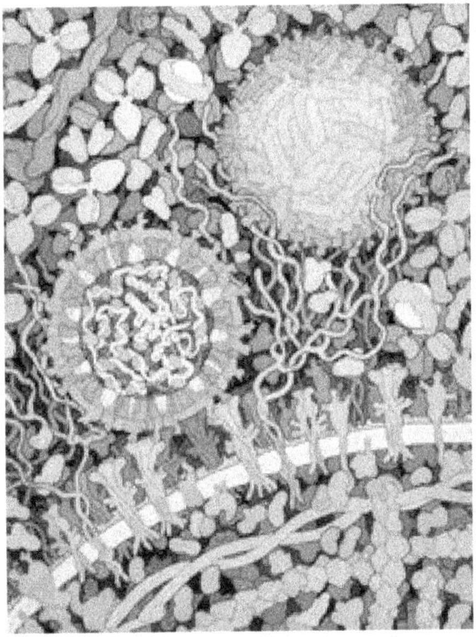

Cross-section of Zika virus, with capsid layer (round structures), membrane layer (lower), and RNA genome (upper and middle)

A positive-sense RNA genome can be directly translated into viral proteins. In other flaviviruses, such as the similarly sized West Nile virus, the RNA genome genes encode seven nonstructural proteins and three structural proteins. The structural proteins encapsulate the virus. The replicated RNA strand is held within a nucleocapsid formed from 12-kDa protein blocks; the capsid is contained within a host-derived membrane modified with two viral glycoproteins. Replication of the viral genome would first require creation of an anti-sense nucleotide strand.

There are two lineages of Zika: the African lineage and the Asian lineage. Phylogenetic studies indicate that the virus spreading in the Americas is a hybrid with 89% identical to African genotypes, yet is closely related to the Asian strain that circulated in French Polynesia during the 2013–2014 outbreak.

CHAPTER TWO: TRANSMISSION

The vertebrate hosts of the virus were primarily monkeys in a so-called enzootic mosquito-monkey-mosquito cycle, with only occasional transmission to humans. Before the current pandemic began in 2007, *Zika* rarely caused recognized *spillover* infections in humans, even in highly enzootic areas. Infrequently, however, other arboviruses have become established as a human disease and spread in a mosquito–human–mosquito cycle, like the yellow fever virus and the dengue fever virus (both *flaviviruses*), and the *chikungunya* virus (a *togavirus)*. Though the reason for the pandemic is unknown, dengue, a related *arbovirus* that infects the same species of mosquito vectors, is known in particular to be intensified by urbanization and globalization.

Mosquito:

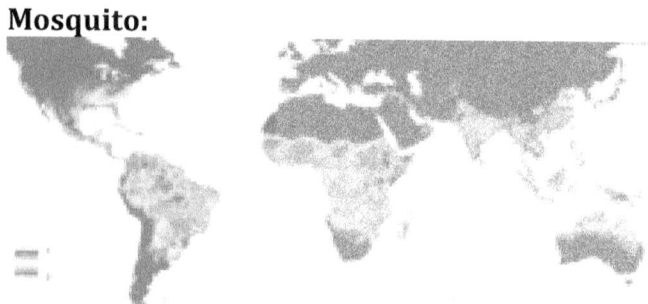

Global *Aedes aegypti* predicted distribution. The map depicts the probability of occurrence.

Zika is primarily spread by the female *Aedes aegypti* mosquito, which is active mostly in the daytime, although researchers have found the virus in common *Culex* house mosquitoes as well. The mosquitos must feed on blood in order to lay eggs. The virus has also been isolated from a number of arboreal mosquito species in the *Aedes* genus, such as *A. africanus*, *A. apicoargenteus*, *A. furcifer*, *A. hensilli*, *A.*

luteocephalus and A. vittatus, with an extrinsic incubation period in mosquitoes of about 10 days.

The true extent of the vectors is still unknown. *Zika* has been detected in many more species of *Aedes,* along with *Anopheles coustani, Mansonia uniformis,* and *Culex perfuscus,* although this alone does not incriminate them as a vector.

Transmission by *A. albopictus,* the tiger mosquito, was reported from a 2007 urban outbreak in Gabon where it had newly invaded the country and become the primary vector for the concomitant *chikungunya* and *dengue* virus outbreaks. There is concern for *autochthonous* infections in urban areas of European countries infested by *A. albopictus* because the first two cases of laboratory-confirmed *Zika* infections imported into Italy were reported from *viremic* travelers returning from French Polynesia.

The potential societal risk of *Zika* can be delimited by the distribution of the mosquito species that transmit it. The global distribution of the most cited carrier of *Zika, A. aegypti,* is expanding due to global trade and travel.

A. aegypti distribution is now the most extensive ever recorded – across all continents including North America and even the European periphery (Madeira, the Netherlands, and the northeastern Black Sea coast).

A mosquito population capable of carrying *Zika* has been found in a Capitol Hill neighborhood of Washington, D. C., and genetic evidence suggests they survived at least four consecutive winters in the region. The study authors conclude that mosquitos are adapting for persistence in a northern climate.

The *Zika* virus appears to be contagious via mosquitoes for around a week after infection. The virus is thought to be infectious for a longer period of time after infection (2 weeks) when transmitted via semen.

Since 2015, news reports have drawn attention to the spread of *Zika* in Latin America and the Caribbean. The countries and territories that have been identified by the Pan American Health Organization as having experienced "local *Zika* virus transmission" are Barbados, Bolivia, Brazil, Colombia, the Dominican Republic, Ecuador, El Salvador, French Guiana, Guadeloupe, Guatemala, Guyana, Haiti, Honduras, Martinique,

Mexico, Panama, Paraguay, Puerto Rico, Saint Martin, Suriname, and Venezuela.

Research into its ecological niche suggests that *Zika* may be influenced to a greater degree by changes in precipitation and temperature than *Dengue*, making it more likely to be confined to tropical areas. However, rising global temperatures would allow for the disease vector to expand their range further north, allowing *Zika* to follow.

Sexual:

Zika can be transmitted from a man or a woman to their sexual partners. As of April 2016 sexual transmission of *Zika* has been documented in six countries – Argentina, Chile, France, Italy, New Zealand and the United States – during the 2015 outbreak.

In 2014, *Zika* capable of growth in lab culture was found in the semen of a man at least two weeks (and possibly up to 10 weeks) after he fell ill with *Zika* fever. In 2011 a study found that a United States biologist who had been bitten many times while studying mosquitoes in Senegal developed symptoms six days after returning home in August 2008, but not before having unprotected intercourse with his wife, who had not been outside the US since 2008. Both husband and wife were confirmed to have *Zika* antibodies, raising awareness of the possibility of sexual transmission. In early February 2016, the *Dallas County Health and Human Services Department* reported that a man from Texas who had not travelled abroad had been infected after his male monogamous sexual partner had anal penetrative sex with him one day before and one day after the onset of symptoms.

As of February 2016, fourteen additional cases of possible sexual transmission have been under investigation, but it remained unknown whether women can transmit *Zika* to their sexual partners. At that time, the understanding of the incidence and duration of shedding in the male genitourinary tract was limited to one case report. Therefore, the *United States Centers for Disease Control and Prevention (CDC)* interim guideline recommended against testing men for purposes of assessing the risk of sexual transmission.

In March 2016, the *CDC* updated its recommendations about length of precautions for couples, and advised that heterosexual couples with men who have confirmed *Zika* fever or symptoms of *Zika* should consider using condoms or not having penetrative sex (i.e., vaginal intercourse, anal intercourse, or fellatio) for at least 6 months after symptoms begin. This includes men who live in—and men who traveled to—areas with *Zika*. Couples with men who traveled to an area with *Zika*, but did not develop symptoms of *Zika*, should consider using condoms or not having sex for at least 8 weeks after their return in order to minimize risk. Couples with men who live in an area with *Zika*, but have not developed symptoms, might consider using condoms or not having sex while there is active *Zika* transmission in the area.

Pregnancy:

The *Zika* virus can spread from an infected mother to her fetus during pregnancy or at delivery.

Blood transfusion:

As of April 2016, two cases of *Zika* transmission through blood transfusions have been reported globally, both from Brazil, after which the

US Food and Drug Administration recommended screening blood donors and deferring high-risk donors for 4 weeks. A potential risk had been suspected based on a blood-donor screening study during the French Polynesian *Zika* outbreak, in which 2.8% or 42 of the donors from November 2013 through February 2014 tested positive for *Zika* RNA and were all asymptomatic at the time of the blood donation. Eleven of the positive donors reported symptoms of *Zika* fever after their donation, but only three of 34 samples grew in culture.

CHAPTER THREE: HISTORY

Virus isolation in monkeys and mosquitoes, 1947:

The virus was first isolated in April 1947 from a rhesus macaque monkey that had been placed in a cage in the Zika Forest of Uganda, near Lake Victoria, by the scientists of the Yellow Fever Research Institute. A second isolation from the mosquito *A. africanus* followed at the same site in January 1948. When the monkey developed a fever, researchers isolated from its serum a "filterable transmissible agent" that was named Zika in 1948.

First evidence of human infection, 1952:

Zika had been known to infect humans from the results of serological surveys in Uganda and Nigeria, published in 1952: Among 84 people of all ages, 50 individuals had antibodies to Zika, and all above 40 years of age were immune. A 1952 research study conducted in India had shown a "significant number" of Indians tested for Zika had exhibited an immune response to the virus, suggesting it had long been widespread within human populations.

It was not until 1954 that the isolation of Zika from a human was published. This came as part of a 1952 outbreak investigation of jaundice suspected to be yellow fever. It was found in the blood of a 10-year-old Nigerian female with a low-grade fever, headache, and evidence of malaria, but no jaundice, who recovered within three days. Blood was injected into the brain of laboratory mice, followed by up to 15 mice passages. The virus from mouse brains was then tested in neutralization tests using rhesus monkey sera specifically immune to Zika. In contrast, no virus was isolated from the blood of two infected adults with fever, jaundice, cough, diffuse joint pains in one and fever, headache, pain behind the eyes and in the joints. Infection was proven by a rise in Zika-specific serum antibodies.

Spread in equatorial Africa and to Asia, 1951–1983:

From 1951 through 1983, evidence of human infection with Zika was reported from other African countries, such as the Central African Republic, Egypt, Gabon, Sierra Leone, Tanzania, and Uganda, as well as in parts of Asia including India, Indonesia, Malaysia, the Philippines, Thailand, Vietnam and Pakistan. From its discovery until 2007, there were only 14 confirmed human cases of Zika infection from Africa and Southeast Asia.

Micronesia, 2007:

In April 2007, the first outbreak outside of Africa and Asia occurred on the island of Yap in the Federated States of Micronesia, characterized by rash, conjunctivitis, and arthralgia, which was initially thought to be dengue, chikungunya, or Ross River disease. Serum samples from patients in the acute phase of illness contained

RNA of Zika. There were 49 confirmed cases, 59 unconfirmed cases, no hospitalizations, and no deaths.

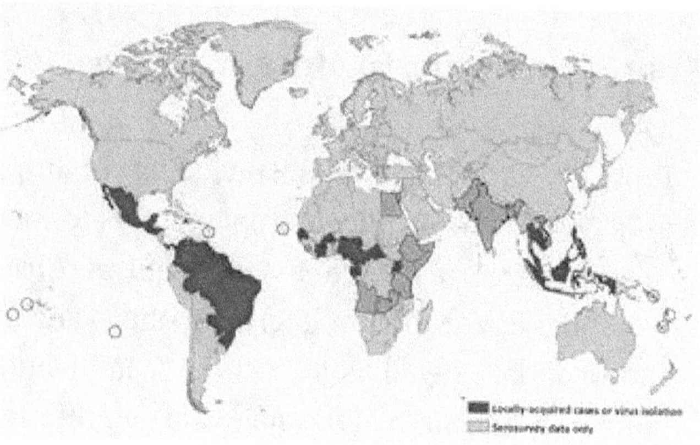

2007 Yap Islands Zika virus outbreak

2013–2014:

Oceania:

Between 2013 and 2014, further epidemics occurred in French Polynesia, Easter Island, the Cook Islands, and New Caledonia.

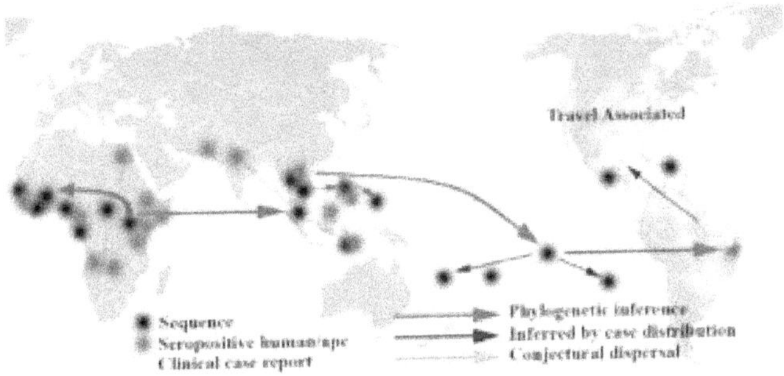

2013–2014 Zika virus outbreaks in Oceania

Other cases:

On 22 March 2016 Reuters reported that Zika was isolated from a 2014 blood sample of an elderly man in Chittagong in Bangladesh as part of a retrospective study.

Americas, 2015–present:

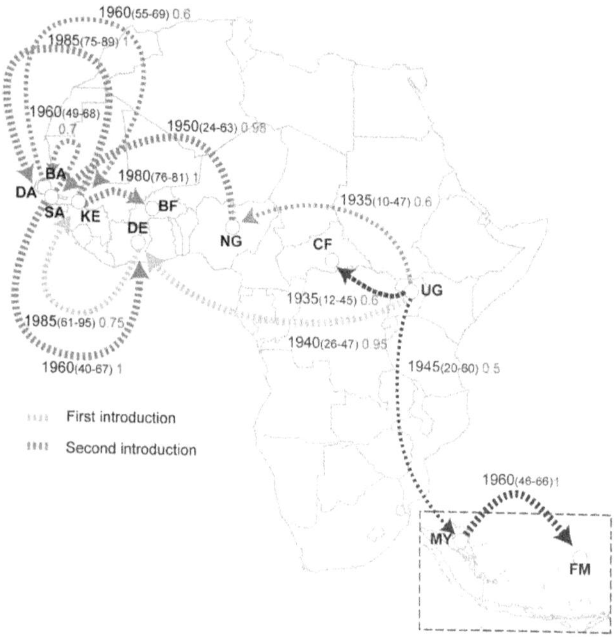

2015–16 Zika virus epidemic

As of early 2016, a widespread outbreak of Zika was ongoing, primarily in the Americas. The outbreak began in April 2015 in Brazil, and has spread to other countries in South America, Central America, Mexico, and the Caribbean. In January 2016, the WHO said the virus was likely to spread throughout most of the Americas by the end of the year; and in February 2016, the WHO declared the cluster of microcephaly and

Guillain–Barré syndrome cases reported in Brazil – strongly suspected to be associated with the Zika outbreak – a Public Health Emergency of International Concern. It is estimated that 1.5 million people have been infected by Zika in Brazil, with over 3,500 cases of microcephaly reported between October 2015 and January 2016.

A number of countries have issued travel warnings, and the outbreak is expected to significantly impact the tourism industry. Several countries have taken the unusual step of advising their citizens to delay pregnancy until more is known about the virus and its impact on fetal development.

With the 2016 Olympics Games set to be hosted in Rio de Janeiro, health officials worldwide have voiced concerns over a potential crisis, both in Brazil and when international athletes and tourists, who may be unknowingly infected, return home and possibly spread the virus. Some researchers speculate that only one or two tourists may be infected during the three week period, or approximately 3.2 infections per 100,000 tourists.

CHAPTER FOUR: PATHOGENESIS

Zika virus replicates in the mosquito's midgut epithelial cells and then its salivary gland cells. After 5–10 days, the virus can be found in the mosquito's saliva, which can then infect humans. If the mosquito's saliva is inoculated into human skin, the virus can infect epidermal keratinocytes, skin fibroblasts in the skin and the Langerhans cells. The pathogenesis of the virus is hypothesized to continue with a spread to lymph nodes and the bloodstream. Flaviviruses generally replicate in the cytoplasm, but Zika antigens have been found in infected cell nuclei.

Zika fever:

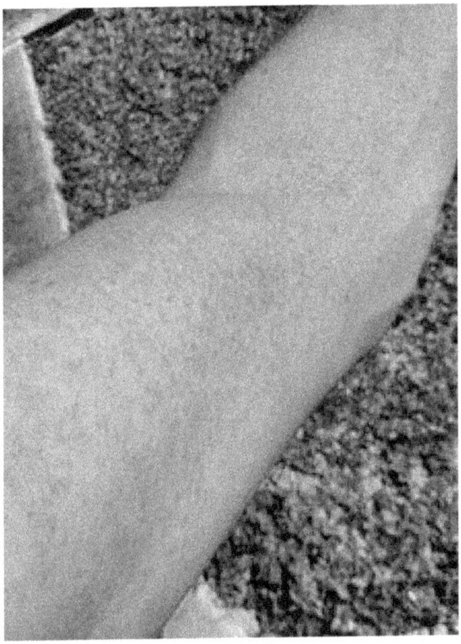

Rash on an arm due to Zika

Zika fever (also known as Zika virus disease) is an illness caused by the Zika virus. Most cases have no symptoms, but when present they are usually mild and can resemble dengue fever. Symptoms may include fever, red eyes, joint pain, headache, and a maculopapular rash. Symptoms generally last less than seven days. It has not caused any reported deaths during the initial infection. Infection during pregnancy causes microcephaly and other brain malformations in some babies. Infections in adults has been linked to Guillain–Barré syndrome (GBS).

Diagnosis is by testing the blood, urine, or saliva for the presence of Zika virus RNA when the person is sick.

Prevention involves decreasing mosquito bites in areas where the disease occurs and proper use of condoms. Efforts to prevent bites include the use of insect repellent, covering much of the body with clothing, mosquito nets, and getting rid of standing water where mosquitoes reproduce.

There is no effective vaccine. Health officials recommended that women in areas affected by the 2015–16 Zika outbreak consider putting off pregnancy and that pregnant women not travel to these areas. While there is no specific treatment, paracetamol (acetaminophen) and rest may help with the symptoms. Admission to hospital is rarely necessary.

Vaccine Development:

Effective vaccines have existed for several viruses of the flaviviridae family, namely yellow fever vaccine, Japanese encephalitis vaccine, and tick-borne encephalitis vaccine, since the 1930s, and for the dengue fever vaccine since the mid-2010s.

WHO experts have suggested that the priority should be to develop inactivated vaccines and other non-live vaccines, which are safe to use in pregnant women and those of childbearing age.

The National Institute of Health (NIH) Vaccine Research Center (U.S.) began work towards developing a vaccine for Zika per a January 2016 report.

Bharat Biotech International (India) reported in early February 2016, that it was working on vaccines for Zika using two approaches: (1) **Recombinant**, involving genetic engineering, and (2) **Inactivated**, where the virus is incapable of reproducing itself but can still trigger an immune response with animal trials of the inactivated version to commence in late February.

As of March 2016, 18 companies and institutions internationally were developing vaccines against Zika, but none had yet reached clinical trials.

The first human trial for a Zika vaccine, a synthetic DNA vaccine (GLS-5700) developed by

Inovio Pharmaceuticals, was approved by the FDA in June 2016. Interim results of the Phase 1 study is expected in later 2016.

CHAPTER FIVE: *AEDES AEGYPTI* VERSUS *AEDES ALBOPICTUS* MOSQUITOS IN THE UNITED STATES

The next pages shows an estimated range of *Aedes aegypti* versus *Aedes albopictus* mosquito infection in the United States, from left to right, as of 2016; this data us based on CDC results.

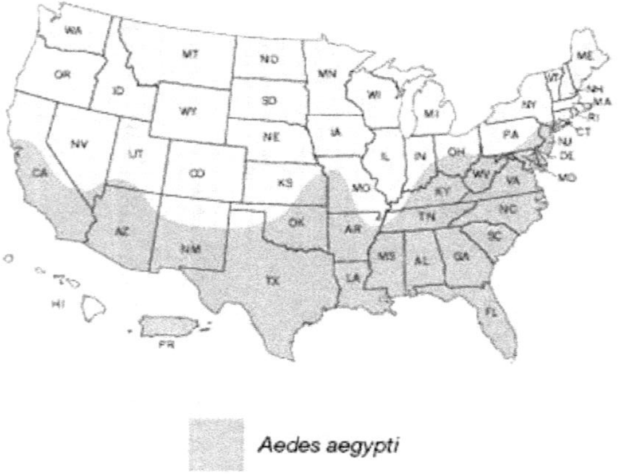
Aedes aegypti

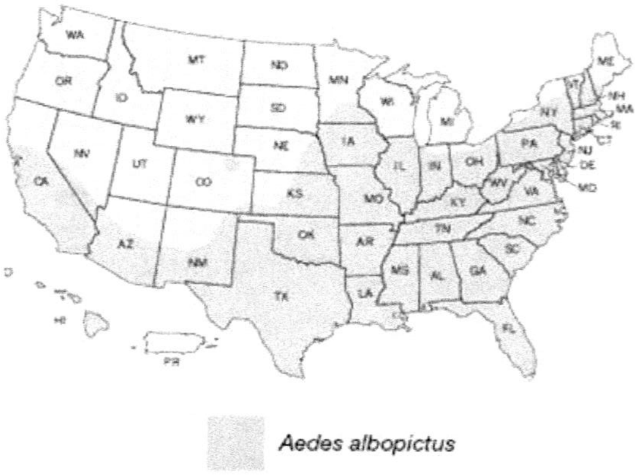
Aedes albopictus

The new estimated range maps have been updated from a variety of published and unpublished sources. These maps show CDC's best estimate of the potential range of *Aedes aegypti* and *Aedes albopictus* in the United States. These maps include areas where mosquitoes are or have been previously found. The maps are **not** meant to represent risk for spread of disease.

Aedes aegypti mosquitoes are more likely to spread viruses like Zika, dengue, chikungunya and other viruses than other types of mosquitoes such as *Aedes albopictus* mosquitoes.

About these mosquitoes:

Aedes aegypti

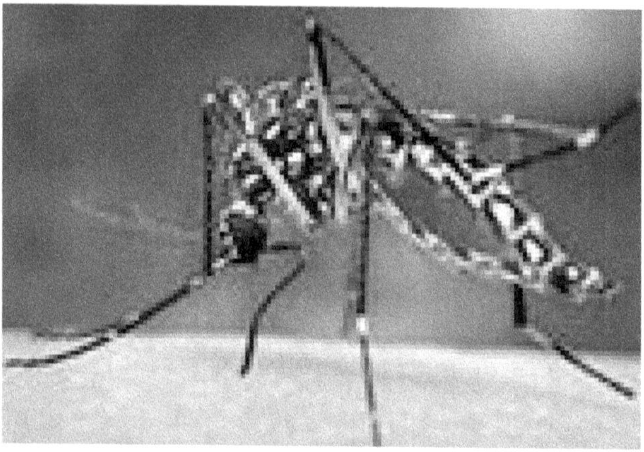

These mosquitoes live in tropical, subtropical, and in some temperate climates.

They are the main type of mosquito that spread Zika, dengue, chikungunya, and other viruses.

Because *Aedes aegypti* mosquitoes live near and prefer to feed on people, they are more likely to spread these viruses than other types of mosquitoes.

Aedes albopictus

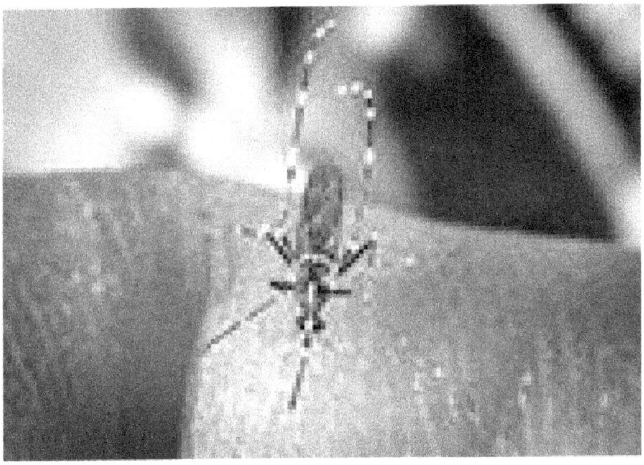

These mosquitoes live tropical, subtropical, and temperate climates, but can live in a broader temperature range and at cooler temperatures than *Aedes aegypti.*

Because these mosquitoes feed on animals as well as people, they are less likely to spread viruses like Zika, dengue, chikungunya and other viruses.

About outbreaks spread by mosquitoes:

Local mosquito-borne Zika virus transmission has been reported in the continental United States.

Many areas in the United States have the type of mosquitoes that can become infected with and spread Zika, chikungunya, and dengue viruses.

Recent outbreaks in the continental United States of chikungunya and dengue, which are spread by the same type of mosquito, have been relatively small and limited to a small area.

Areas with past outbreaks of chikungunya and dengue are considered at higher risk for Zika. These include U.S. territories like Puerto Rico, the U.S. Virgin Islands, and Guam. Local outbreaks have also been reported in parts of Hawaii, Florida, and Texas.

Aedes aegypti or *Aedes albopictus* mosquitoes can cause an outbreak, if all of the following happens:

1. People get infected with a virus (like Zika, dengue, or chikungunya).
2. An *Aedes aegypti* or *Aedes albopictus* mosquito bites an infected person during the first week of infection when the virus can be found in the person's blood.
3. The infected mosquito lives long enough for the virus to multiply and for the mosquito to bite another person.
4. The cycle continues multiple times to start an outbreak.

Scientists at CDC advise people in the United States to protect themselves from Zika and other viruses spread by mosquitoes

The best way to prevent Zika and other viruses spread through mosquito bites is to take steps to prevent mosquito bites, especially if pregnant:

1. Wear long-sleeved shirts and long pants.
2. Stay in places with air conditioning and use window and door screens to keep mosquitoes outside.
3. Use Environmental Protection Agency (EPA)-registered insect repellents with one of the following active ingredients: DEET, picaridin, IR3535, oil of lemon eucalyptus, or para-menthane-diol. When used as directed, EPA-registered insect repellents are proven safe and effective, even for pregnant and breastfeeding women.
4. Treat clothing with permethrin or purchase permethrin-treated items.

CHAPTER SIX:

ZIKA INFECTIONS IN THE UNITED STATES

Since March 10, 2016, the number of Zika virus cases reported to the CDC has risen from 193 cases in the United States to 258, and from 174 cases in the U.S. territories to 286, for a total of 544.

Of the 258 travel-associated cases in the states, 18 are in pregnant women and six were sexually transmitted. The March 2016 report is the first report in which the CDC specified sexually transmitted cases and cases in pregnant women.

There are still no reports of locally acquired cases in the United States, but the number of locally acquired cases in the U.S. territories has jumped from 173 to 283, according to the most recent CDC data. Of the locally-acquired cases in the territories, 35 are in pregnant women.

Zika cases in the United States

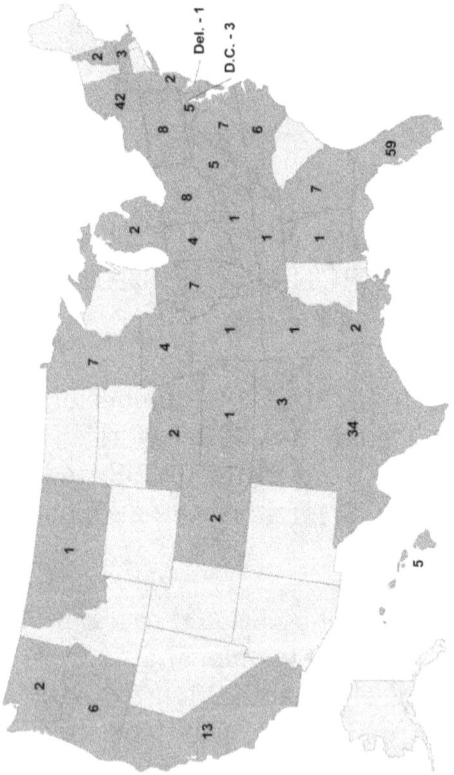

Not pictured: Fourteen locally-acquired cases have been reported in the American Samoa, 259 cases in Puerto Rico and 10 cases in the U.S. Virgin Islands. There has also been two travel-associated case reported in Puerto Rico and one in the U.S. Virgin Islands.

CHAPTER SEVEN:
THE ROCKEFELLER FOUNDATION IS SELLING THE ZIKA VIRUS ONLINE

The virus has been around for over 60 years and is marketed by two companies: LGC Standards (in the UK) and ATCC (in the US).

Here is a link to the site in the United States, by the ATCC Corporation:
https://www.atcc.org/Products/All/VR-84.aspx?geo_country=us#history

The following are what are found on each of the tabs of the preceding link, beginning with:

HISTORY:

Name of Depositor	J. Casals, Rockefeller Foundation
Source	Blood from experimental forest sentinel rhesus monkey, Uganda, 1947
Year of Origin	1947
References	Dick GW, Kitchen SF, and Haddow AJ. Zika Virus. I. Isolations and Serological Specificity. Trans R Soc Trop Med Hyg 46: 509-520, 1952. PubMed: 12995440 Zhu Z, et al. Comparative genomic analysis of pre-epidemic and epidemic Zika virus strains for virological factors potentially associated with the rapidly expanding epidemic. Emerg Microbes

Infect 5: e22, 2016.

GENERAL INFORMATION:

Classification *Flaviviridae, Flavivirus*

Agent Zika virus

Strain MR 766 (Original)

Biosafety Level 2

Biosafety classification is based on U.S. Public Health Service Guidelines, it is the responsibility of the customer to ensure that their facilities comply with biosafety regulations for their own country.

Product Format freeze-dried

Storage Conditions -70°C or colder

CHARACTERISTICS:

Comments	The depositor reports that ATCC® VR-84™ can agglutinate goose and chicken RBC, and that this strain is non-pathogenic for hamster, guinea pig, or rabbit. Accidental infection has occurred in laboratory personnel The lyophilized culture is stable at 4°C, and should be stored at -70°C or colder once rehydrated
Effect on Host	Paralysis and death

CULTURE METHOD:

Recommended Host	Suckling mouse
Growth Conditions	**Recommendations for Infection:** Inoculate intracerebrally into suckling mice. Resuspend 20% sMb with 7.5% BSA in PBS. **Incubation**: 5-7 days

SPECIFICATIONS:

Effect on Host Paralysis and death

DOCUMENTATION:

Permits:

These permits may be required for shipping this product:

Customer Acceptance of Responsibility, ATCC Form 62 required for distribution.

Customers located in the state of Hawaii will need to contact the Hawaii Department of Agriculture to determine if an Import Permit is required. A copy of the permit or documentation that a permit is not required must be sent to ATCC in advance of shipment.

FAQs:

1. What is Zika virus
   Zika virus is a single-stranded RNA virus of the Flaviviridae family, genus Flavivirus (which also includes the Dengue, and West Nile Viruses). Zika virus is transmitted to humans primarily ...

Date Updated: 3/3/2016

2. <u>Is Zika a new virus</u>

No. According to the CDC, Zika previously has been reported in tropical Africa, Southeast Asia, and the Pacific Islands. In May 2015, the Pan American Health Organization (PAHO) issued an alert r...

Date Updated: 2/5/2016

3. <u>Does ATCC distribute the Zika virus</u>

Yes, Zika virus (ATCC® VR-84™) strain MR766 has been distributed by ATCC since 1953. The virus is available through ATCC, and our designated Source of VR-84 Zika The virus was deposited into ATCC by Dr. Jordi Casals of the Rockefeller Foundation Virus Laboratory in 1953. The original source was isolated in 1947 from the blood of an experimental forest sen...

Date Updated: 2/5/2016

4. <u>Obtaining Zika</u>

Zika virus is classified as a biological safety level (BSL) 2 pathogen. In order to request Zika virus from ATCC, requestors and their institutions must demonstrate they have appropriate faciliti...

Date Updated: 2/5/2016

5. Safety of Zika shipments

All ATCC shipments meet all domestic and global regulatory requirements for packaging, labeling and shipping of hazardous biological materials.

Date Updated: 2/5/2016

ATCC even has two forms of the Zika Virus the accidental "scientific researcher," or maybe not so accidental "scientific researcher" can purchase: A more upscale, more expensive one; or if you're in a real big hurry to "do your Zika research," there is a less expensive one:

Classification: ***Flaviviridae, Flavivirus***

Zika virusATCC® VR-84™

Product format: freeze-dried

For-Profit: $516.00 Non-Profit: $430.00

Qty:

Add to Cart

RELATED PRODUCTS

Zika virus (ATCC® VR-1838™)

Add to

frozen 1.0 mL

For-Profit: $354.00 Non-Profit: $295.00

And when *I* clicked on the more upscale one, of course, it put it in my shopping cart, and was willing, able, and ready to take my credit card, no questions asked. I thought I needed a permit? Imagine that. It appears that anyone with a credit card can purchase the Zika virus from ATCC, whose major sponsor, donor, endowment, funding comes from The Rockefeller Foundation.

1 Item added to cart

VR-84

Zika virus (ATCC® VR-84™)

Quantity: 1

Biosafety Level: 2

Price: $516.00

Cart summary (1 item)

Subtotal:$516.00

View entire cart

Proceed to Checkout Continue Shopping

Apparently the Zika virus started in Uganda back in 1947 where is was found in monkeys.

Blood samples were taken from the monkeys and freeze-dried and are now on sale, presumably for researchers to use in vaccine testing.

According to **Aangirfan**: *The Uganda/East African Virus Research Institute, in Entebbe, Uganda, was established in 1936 by the* ***Rockefeller Foundation.***

The institute has a field station at the ***Zika Forest*** *near Entebbe.*

In 1947 scientists placed a rhesus macaque in a cage in the Zika Forest, near the institute in Entebbe, Uganda.

The monkey developed a fever, and researchers isolated from its serum a transmissible agent that was first described as Zika virus in 1952.

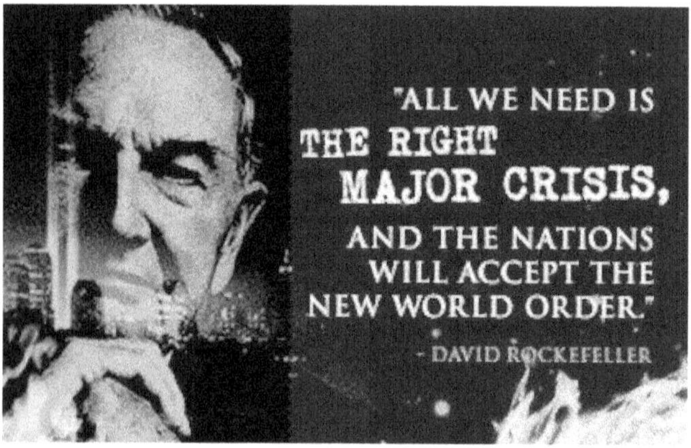
"ALL WE NEED IS
THE RIGHT
MAJOR CRISIS,
AND THE NATIONS
WILL ACCEPT THE
NEW WORLD ORDER."
- DAVID ROCKEFELLER

CHAPTER EIGHT:
THE ZIKA VIRUS, BILL GATES, AND DEPOPULATION

The Zika virus was first discovered in 1947 throughout Africa and southern Asia, so this is nothing new. Eyebrows were raised in 2013 when small outbreaks and individual cases were officially documented in Africa, the western pacific, and the Americas. The Antimedia ... and media reports that "Brazil is now considered the epicenter of the Zika outbreak, which coincides with at least 4,000 reports of babies born with microcephaly just since October." Microcephaly is a birth defect associated with a shrunken brain.

The World Health Organization stated the Zika virus could potentially pose a bigger threat to global health. With that, President Obama called for a massive research effort to develop a vaccine for solutions and future prevention.

The Zika virus had never been a threat to the global population before, so what really happened between 2010 and 2015?

The Mirror reported on the Zika virus where they asked if the virus was possibly spread through the release of genetically modified (GM) mosquitoes. If so, then the case backfired dramatically, from a public perspective, or was it so accidental afterall:

"The insects were engineered by biotechnology experts to combat the spread of dengue fever and other diseases and released into the general population of Brazil in 2012...up to 1.5 million people are now thought to be affected by the virus"

According to Infowars a startling coincidence has been made in relation to Bill Gates and his GM mosquitoes.

"In 2010, the Bill & Melinda Gates Foundation funded Australian researchers to release GM mosquitoes infected with a bacterium."

That same year, Bill Gates admitted he believed in population reduction:

"The world today has 6.8 billion people; that's headed up to about 9 billion," he said during the TED 2010 Conference. "Now if we do a really great job on new vaccines, health care, reproductive health services, we lower that by perhaps 10 or 15 percent."

Trinfinity8 reports on the darker untold story behind the suspected GM mosquito scheme, writing:

"The mosquito Gates released was likely to be a long-term dream of his he had for forced birth control and forced vaccinations, which he has been working on since 2003.

In the forced vaccination scenario, the mosquitoes are genetically programmed to produce the "vaccine" permanently once released into the environment, so they would not have to release new mosquitoes EVER again. Their effects would simply become part of nature.

This means that at some time in your life you and everyone else is bound to be bitten by a mosquito created by Bill Gates."

The Gates Foundation is about benefiting big business, and according to Trinfinity8, in 2015 the Vanderbilt Vaccine Program received a grant for $307,000 dollars from the Bill & Melinda Gates Foundation to study the immune responses of pregnant women who received the mandatory Tdap (Tetanus, Diptheria, Pertussis) vaccine Brazilian minister of health put into regulation, 2014. "None of the raw results could be found."

Infowars also held an interview with International law professor Francis A. Boyle, who drafted the Biological Weapons Anti-Terrorism Act of 1989, where he revealed the Zika virus was "souped up as a bio weapon by world governments and non-government organizations."

Could there be a chance that Bill Gates may have "souped up" the Zika virus for himself?

Chapter eight was referenced completely through the following sources: TheAntimedia; Mirror; Trinfinity8; Infowars; and Truthandaction.

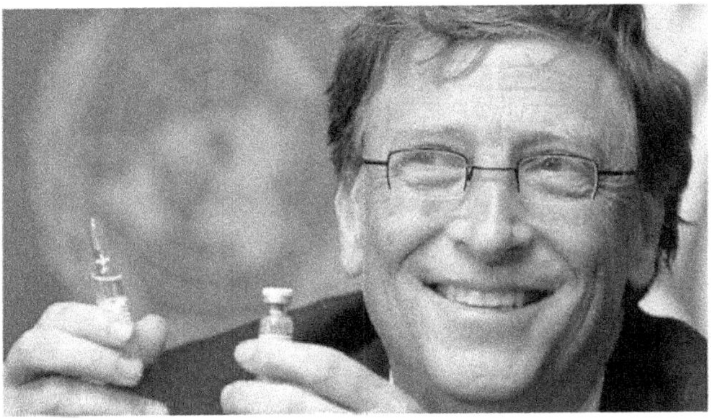

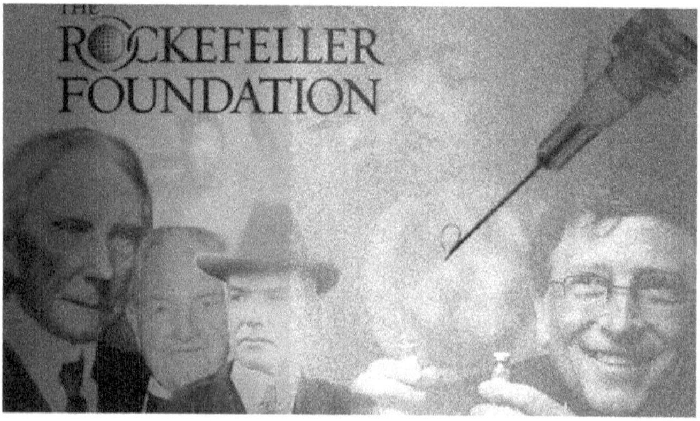

ROCKEFELLER
FOUNDATION

CHAPTER NINE: RUSSIA ACCUSES BILL GATES OF DEPOPULATION

In one of the most controversial yet underplayed stories of the year so far Russia has accused Microsoft owner and Billionaire Bill Gates, of "Engineering the believed 'Bioweapon' Zika Virus:" The Zika virus is a deadly bioweapon that is using GMO (genetically modified) mosquitos to spread around the planet 'future diseases' according to an intriguing Kremlin report apparently – And the finger of blame is being pointed directly at Bill

Gates for the responsibility of this vile disease/weapon.

Apparently the destructive bioweapon was developed by the Microsoft owner alongside other members of the Elite world to achieve his very self-confessed Illuminati goal of "depopulating" the worlds masses, a term Bill Gates, himself developed.

Already there is a leaked highly confidential Foreign Intelligence Service (SVR) report that has been read by senior sources in the Kremlin, which supposedly revealed that the Zika virus was actually "cooked up as a bioweapon" by certain "world governments and non-government ELITE organizations." It is understood the chief non-government organization behind the Zika virus is Bill Gates' own **Bill & Melinda Gates Foundation**.

It has been confirmed that the Russian leader President Putin is said to be angered. There have also been meetings in the past week regarding banning Gates from the Russian

Federation, as well as plans to protect the human race from the "world government created bioweapon." Russia has for a log while stated that illuminati are planning some kind of worldwide attack on us all.

*"GMOs are humanity's mortal enemy and these sick b****** won't be happy until most of us are dead.... Western powers are in their final death throes, thrashing about and clutching at straws, using the last weapons in their arsenal of dirty tricks against humanity. We must not allow these GMO serial killers to poison our children," stated a Russian source close to Putin.*

Russia has recently also said that they believe the US and its allies are responsible behind the making of the terrorist army in the middle east, who call themselves the Islamic State (ISIS/Daesh). Conspiracy theories appear to be coming true it seems, according to Russia.

It was back in 2010, when the **Bill & Melinda Gates Foundation** funded Australian research scientists to release GMO mosquitoes infected with a bacterium. This very same year, Bill Gates even confessed he wanted to depopulate the world – which is THE key Illuminati goal:

"The world today has 6.8 billion people; that's headed up to about 9 billion," he said during the invitation-only 2010 TED Conference.

"Now if we do a really great job on new vaccines, health care, reproductive health services, we lower that by perhaps 10 or 15 percent," Bill Gates said.

And now it appears that those bacterium-infected GMO mosquitoes which were apparently co-created by Bill Gates back in 2010, are wreaking havoc in the Americas – with the whole planet now at risk, according to the World Health Organization (WHO).

WHO is now convening an Emergency Committee under International Health Regulations concerning the 'explosive' spread of the Zika virus throughout the Americas. The virus reportedly has the potential to reach pandemic proportions — possibly around the globe. But understanding why this outbreak happened is vital to stopping it from spreading across the planet – The finger of blame is now being pointed directly at the richest man in the world, but what can be done about this war crime against humanity?

Could this be the start of something much bigger, perhaps a war against **U.I.P SUMMARY** – At first this story could be deemed as over the top, but is it really? Remember Ebola and how that exploded onto the scene and then suddenly fizzled out? Perhaps that was the first FAILED attempt to de-populate and this disease is a far more serious threat than what we have been reading about in the news.

Or perhaps this is just another false flag event to distract us from something else going on....but what?

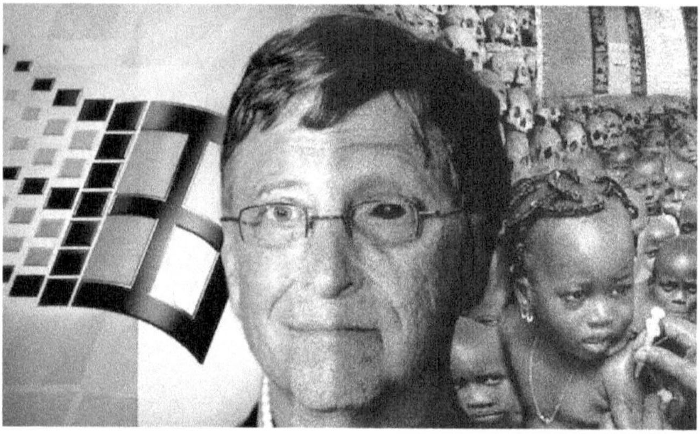

CHAPTER TEN: LONDON ACCUSES BILL GATES OF DEPOPULATION

In a recent interview with the *London Telegraph*, Bill Gates has now claimed that his Foundation's massive push for vaccination is not just an exercise in philanthropy but that it is, in fact, "God's work."

Gates, who, according to the Telegraph, is worth an estimated $65 billion, is now dedicating his life to the "eradication of poliomyelitis," or, at least he is dedicating himself to the vaccination program allegedly aimed at achieving these ends.

As reported by the Telegraph,

"My wife and I had a long dialogue about how we were going to take the wealth that we're lucky enough to have and give it back in a way that's most impactful to the world," he says.

"Both of us worked at Microsoft and saw that if you take innovation and smart people, the ability to measure what's working, that you can pull together some pretty dramatic things.

"We're focused on the help of the poorest in the world, which really drives you into vaccination. You can actually take a disease and get rid of it altogether, like we are doing with polio."

Yet, eradicating polio through a massive vaccination program may be easier said than done writes Neil Tweedie of the Telegraph. "There is another, sinister obstacle: the propagation by Islamist groups of the belief that polio vaccination is a front for covert sterilisation and other western evils. Health workers in Pakistan have paid with their lives for involvement in the programme."

To this question, Gates responded with seemingly atypical religious zeal, noted by Tweedie in the published article. “It’s not going to stop us succeeding,” says Gates.

“It does force us to sit down with the Pakistan government to renew their commitments, see what they’re going to do in security and make changes to protect the women who are doing God’s work and getting out to these children and delivering the vaccine.”

Indeed, the religious tone of Gates during the course of the interview may seem confusing to Tweedie, but the nature of Gates’ work could very well be described as a religion. Thus, the fact that it finds itself in direct confrontation with another religion – the Islamist groups that Tweedie speaks of – is of no real consequence to Gates as his solution is to dutifully press forward.

Yet, before readers write off the vaccine resisters solely as Muslim fundamentalists, many of the individuals opposing vaccination have a very good reason to be skeptical. Especially those that believe Gates' vaccine push is geared more toward sterilization and population reduction than about life extension and better health conditions.

After all, it was Bill Gates himself who stated as much publicly when he said, "The world today has 6.8 billion people... that's headed up to about 9 billion. Now if we do a really great job on new vaccines, health care, reproductive health services, we could lower that by perhaps 10 or 15 percent."

Add this to Gates' statement, is the fact that, time and again, international vaccination programs have ended disastrously for third world nations. Case in point: the recent Meningitis vaccine program that resulted in the paralysis of at least 50 African children and a subsequent cover-up operation by the government of Chad. This large number of adverse events occurred in one small village alone, leaving many to wonder what the rates of side effects might be on an international scale.

Even more concerning is the fact that paralysis rates have flourished in countries where Gates' polio vaccine, the one he is dedicating his life to, have been administered the most. Indeed, nowhere is this any more apparent than in India.

But the real story is that while polio has statistically disappeared from India, there has been a huge spike in cases of non-polio acute flaccid paralysis (NPAFP)– the very types of crippling problems it had hoped would disappear with polio but which had instead flourished from a new cause.

There were 47,500 cases of non-polio paralysis reported in 2011, the same year India was declared "polio-free," according to Dr. Vashisht and Dr. Puliyel. Further, the available data shows that the incidents tracked back to areas were doses of thc polio vaccine were frequently administered. The national rate of NPAFP in India is 25-35 times the international average.

In addition to this data, it appears that the polio vaccines are themselves the leading cause of polio paralysis in India. In relation to the flawed data reported by the Polio Global Eradication Initiative which attempts to minimize the numbers of both vaccine-induced cases of polio paralysis and polio in general, Sayer Ji remarks.

According to the Polio Global Eradication Initiative's own statistics there were 42 cases of wild-type polio (WPV) reported in India in 2010, indicating that vaccine-induced cases of polio paralysis (100-180 annually) outnumber wild-type cases by a factor of 3-4. Even if we put aside the important question of whether or not the PGEI is accurately differentiating between wild and vaccine-associated polio cases in their statistics, we still must ask ourselves: Should not the real-world effects of immunization, both good and bad, be included in PGEI's measurement of success? For the dozens of Indian children who develop vaccine-induced paralysis every year, the PGEI's recent declaration of India as nearing "polio free" status, is not only disingenuous, but could be considered an attempt to minimize their obvious liability in having transformed polio from a natural disease vector into a man-made (iatrogenic) one.

Gates' polio vaccines have likewise been blamed for deaths and disabilities in neighboring Pakistan, with offices of the government in that country even recommending that the vaccines be suspended.

In India, doctors heavily criticized the program not only for the heavy cost to human health and quality of life but also the massive financial burden hoisted upon the state. This is because the program was only partially funded by the Global Alliance for Vaccines and Immunizations, which is itself partnered with the World Health Organization, **Bill and Melinda Gates Foundation, the Rockefeller Foundation**, World Bank, and United Nations.

The doctors criticized the GAVI-alliance by stating,

"The Indian government finally had to fund this hugely expensive programme, which cost the country 100 times more than the value of the initial grant."

From India's perspective the exercise has been extremely costly both in terms of human suffering and in monetary terms. It is tempting to speculate what could have been achieved if the $2.5 billion spent on attempting to eradicate polio, were spent on water and sanitation and routine immunization.

The doctors continue by stating, ". . . . . the polio eradication programme epitomizes nearly everything that is wrong with donor funded 'disease specific' vertical projects at the cost of investments in community-oriented primary health care (horizontal programmes) . . . . .

. . . . .This is a startling reminder of how initial funding and grants from abroad distort local priorities."

Indeed, as the doctors assert, one cannot vaccinate away disease like polio. Apart from the fact that there has never been a study conducted which proves a vaccine either safe or effective that was not connected to a drug company or a vaccine maker, the so-called cure, if it comes under the guise of a vaccine, may well be as bad if not worse than the disease itself.

Again, Sayer Ji writes,

Polio underscores the need for a change in the way we look at so-called "vaccine preventable" diseases as a whole. In most people with a healthy immune system, a poliovirus infection does not even generate symptoms. Only rarely does the infection produce minor symptoms, e.g. sore throat, fever, gastrointestinal disturbances, and influenza-like illness. In only 3% of infections does virus gain entry to the central nervous system, and then, in only 1-5 in 1000 cases does the infection progress to paralytic disease.

Due to the fact that polio spreads through the fecal-oral route (i.e. the virus is transmitted from the stool of an infected person to the mouth of another person through a contaminated object, e.g. utensil) focusing on hygiene, sanitation and proper nutrition (to support innate immunity) is a logical way to prevent transmission in the first place, as well as reducing morbidity associated with an infection when it does occur.

Instead, a large portion of the world's vaccines are given to the Third World as "charity," when the underlying conditions of economic impoverishment, poor nutrition, chemical exposures, and socio-political unrest are never addressed.

The fact is that the root cause of diseases like polio are not a lack of vaccination but poor sanitation standards, poverty, lower living standards, chemical pollution, and lack of proper nutrition. If money were spent correcting these ills, as opposed to providing ineffective (in their stated purposes) and dangerous vaccinations, then polio and many other such diseases could indeed be eradicated.

In the end, the answer is about raising living standards, reducing pollution, increasing knowledge and access to proper nutrition and clean drinking water – not chemical and virus-laden needles. Perhaps this method could be more accurately described as "God's work."

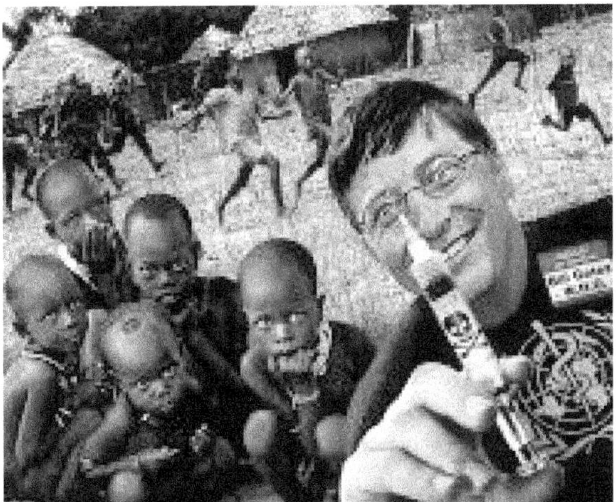

REFERENCES

1. http://hellopoetry.com/poem/1515375/armageddon-or-not/

2. https://en.wikipedia.org/wiki/Zika_virus

3. http://www.npr.org/sections/health-shots/2016/05/17/478251289/who-should-be-worried-about-zika-and-what-should-they-do

4. http://www.cdc.gov/zika/vector/range.html

5. http://www.beckershospitalreview.com/quality/infographic-where-in-the-us-have-zika-cases-been-reported-march-18-update.html

6. http://yournewswire.com/zika-virus-for-sale-online/

7. http://www.truthandaction.org/zika-virus-bill-gates-depopulation/

8. https://www.atcc.org/Products/All/VR-84.aspx?geo_country=us#history

9. https://en.wikipedia.org/wiki/ATCC_(company)

10. http://www.ufointernationalproject.com/latest-news/russia-accuses-bill-gates-for-engineering-the-zika-virus-as-a-de-population-weapon/

11. http://www.activistpost.com/2013/01/bill-gates-says-global-vaccination.html

12. https://www.mosquitosquad.com/zika/

ABOUT THE AUTHOR

Gwendolyn Olmsted, MBA, the former Washington DC microbiologist and research scientist, who conducted graduate level research at major universities as well as United States federal governmental facilities, moved to Florida in 2010. She has a Bachelor's and Master's degree in Business Finance, as well as a second Bachelor's and Master's degree in Environmental Sciences & Sustainability from both private and public universities. Ms. Olmsted has also been employed by the United States Air Force in the early 1990's, stationed in the United Kingdom as well as other locations unable to be disclosed, with an Honorable Discharge. Married to a corporate Washington DC attorney, with children, Gwendolyn now writes stories from the Docu-Eroticamentary, Investigative True Crime, Biographical, Documentary, and Investigative Journalism genres.

OTHER BOOKS WRITTEN BY THE SAME AUTHOR

The Evolution of Ebola

Initially not discovered until 1976 in Sudan, Africa, the Ebola virus was named after the Ebola River near where its first outbreak occurred. Belgian doctor Peter Piot, a 27-year-old scientist and medical school graduate training as a clinical microbiologist, was sent to the region nearly forty years ago to find out why people were dying of a mysterious illness. He uncovered the Ebola virus, yet averted his attention to the virus of the hour, AIDS upon return, so his research abruptly stopped on Ebola. Now Director of the London School of Hygiene and Tropical Medicine, he discusses the initial 1976 strain of Ebola and how it has evolved into the 2014 strain it is today. Virology, epidemiology and outbreaks, Reston and Marburg virus comparisons, research and vaccines, and current death count and outlook are also examined in this handy survival guide to the 2014 Ebola Virus Disease (EBOV) pandemic.

Eight Weeks in May

Based on a true story, *Eight Weeks in May* is a docu-erotica account concerning the manipulative struggles regarding the intricate maneuvers required to survive the legal system in early twenty-first century America, each move carefully calculated, anticipated, and remarkably predictable; predictable like balancing a chemical Redox (reduction-oxidation) equation in a university inorganic chemistry laboratory. Sometimes, though, and always when least expected, the unpredictable happens. Unusually unpredictable is the unstable connection between two courtroom participants, much like reactants in a chemical equation, that when combined produce volatile expectations. A pathway toward erotic fantasies turned realities form as one outlandish scheme bridges into the next, each one building on the last, that terminate with electric and detonating results. Gwendolyn, the former Washington DC microbiologist, whose employs expanded into the federal levels finds herself in a situation where she is misunderstood, wrongly accused of debilitatingly mental illnesses, abandoned, and can't seem to get her bearings straight as she is forced into a position of persuading her most precious of causes; Rob, on the other hand is a district attorney, whose obscured sickingly sweet demeanor and occasional horn-dog tendencies finally catches up to his own exploits, that when the chemical equation called Rob and Gwendolyn finally combine, the most volatile, magnetic, unpredictable and electrical results ever expected are yielded producing the most erotic equation ever known in existence. Inspired by state of Florida, Pinellas County, state's attorney assistant Rob Hauser, III, who stalked Gwendolyn for over one year.

The Pity Date

also published as

American Cockthief

Once upon a time, there was a story of a little girl, a little girl, who was poor, conniving.... scheming, and was willing to do anything to pull herself out of the trailer park she grew up in, anyway that she knew how. That little girl was named Anna Marie Patton. Through lies, manipulations, and some serious cock-sucking techniques, she landed herself a job in the *Guardian ad Litum's* office of Pinellas County, Florida. Because you see, although she did not care about the welfare of the little children, with her bachelor's degree being in Animal Sciences, her position in the *Guardian ad Litum's* Department was the perfect place to meet an attorney, and not just any attorney would do---a district attorney. Follow the nefarious, heinous, corruptive, and spellbinding tactics of one Anna Marie Patton, as she takes advantage of Pinellas County State's Attorney Department's newest hire, Robert Hauser, III, by casting her spells into this mismatched relationship, culminating in their ill-fated October 2007 marriage, as demonstrated by his many girlfriends, his other relationships, and his happiness being ransacked by Anna's lecherous ways, continuing well past their fallacious wedding.

Based on a true story: Yes, people like this really do exist, as some would say, ***only in Florida***.

Sex in Florida

also published as

American Sociopath

Internet dating, a common social affliction of early twenty-first century America, wasn't supposed to involve a long-term commitment. It's purpose, for men was to be for sex, usually in a no-strings-attached arrangement, and anything short of a statutory way to get prostitutionalized sex, legally, and for free. Its purpose for women was to build a relationship with a man of a much higher caliber than a woman would normally meet throughout her day-to-day lifestyle habits. With women on average making significantly less money than men per year, along with that comes meeting men that make as little as they do, because access to higher paid men is not available to women making very little money. With the dawn of Internet dating, came a way for upper class men to meet, although not always lower class women, at least underpaid women, sometimes twentyfold less, as in the case of Christopher and Gwendolyn. Sex in Florida is the true story, written in docu-eroticamentary format, of how an upper class man, Christopher Michaels, found the unexpected love from an underpaid, way overeducated, yet raised upper middle class, woman, environmental scientist, and former Washington DC microbiologist, named Gwendolyn Olmsted. A whirlwind romance develops, evolves, and flourishes, as days lead to weeks, and weeks lead to months, until one day...

The *Sidebar* series

One would not expect to find love inside a courtroom of law, especially between a States Attorney and the defendant he is prosecuting. From the moment Nicholas saw Gwendolyn on the Internet, he could not stop obsessing over her: He invaded all aspects of her life, for over a year and a half, building, wanting, yearning, to finally meet her, until one day, the day he finally met her, engaged her, villainized her .... and seduced her -- in a court of law. Although Gwendolyn didn't know what she was walking into that day, when she had made a required courtroom appearance, from what she initially thought had started out as random Internet dating turned into one of the wildest, salacious, impassioned, seductive, and carnal exploits Gwendolyn had ever fulfilled for Nicholas in his entire life.

belonged to, like there is today. There are no more district attorneys, only state run attorneys that decide the direction of each defendant's fate. The only problem is, sometimes states attorneys commit crimes too. Christopher Martin, a state's attorney assigned to District 2, had the misfortune of being caught killing his wife. Yet his punishment is something completely unexpected and not at all what it is expected to be. But then again, the year is 2555.

Marilyn Monroe: The Live-in Housekeeper did it

The untimely death of one of the most recognized faces who had ever graced Hollywood, Marilyn Monroe, has led to more than one theory surrounding her unsolved departure from the world, the causes, what lead up to it, and contrary to popular belief, The Kennedy's had nothing to do with the death of Marilyn Monroe.

It was the live-in housekeeper, Eunice Murray, whose hand, acting alone, and independently, killed Marilyn, in her sleep, while she was tranquilizing in the seclusion and solitude of her own bedroom in the early evening of August 4th, 1962. Even up until the very day Eunice died in March 1994, no one had ever interviewed her even once .... as a potential suspect.

Marilyn Monroe: The Live-in Housekeeper did it, exploits the evidence and reasoning that points to how and why live-in housekeeper, Eunice Murray, who acting alone, and independently robbed us, Marilyn, and the rest of the world, of perhaps the greatest screen siren of the twentieth century: Marilyn Monroe.

First Place in Short, Short story category at Bay Pines 2016 writing competition

Running on the Luck of my Heart: The Horace Greasley Story

Based on a true story comes a timeless tale of true love, even in the harshest of times. A British Prisoner of War (POW) from the near on-set of his enlistment in World War II, Horace Greasley was caught by the Nazis in May 1940 in the French Countryside where he was working on a railway actually, after a mere five weeks. After a ten week march to the first of two concentration camps he would be confined to for the next five years, he encountered a German woman, seventeen-year-old Rosa Rauchbach, for whom his love and addiction to, would not only save himself, yet enable his comrades to survive under the harsh and cruel conditions of the Nazi prison camps. Against all odds, his love and devotion to Rosa Rauchbach motivated him to escape from his POW prison camp just to be with her, only to return some two-hundred times, undetected, to bring food and supplies to his comrades empowering their survival. ***Running on the Luck of my Heart: The Horace Greasley Story*** is the true story of how one man's love for a young woman on the wrong side of the war saved not only his life, yet the lives of hundreds more.

Available at:

Gwendolyn Olmsted's author page on Amazon.com

www.ingramcontent.com/pod-product-compliance
Lightning Source LLC
Chambersburg PA
CBHW060404190526
45169CB00002B/748
9781536876390